DIABETIC VEGETARIAN MEAL PLAN FOR BEGINNERS

BEGINNERS

A Beginner's Guide to Healthy Eating

By Mia Bennett

COPYRIGHT PAGE

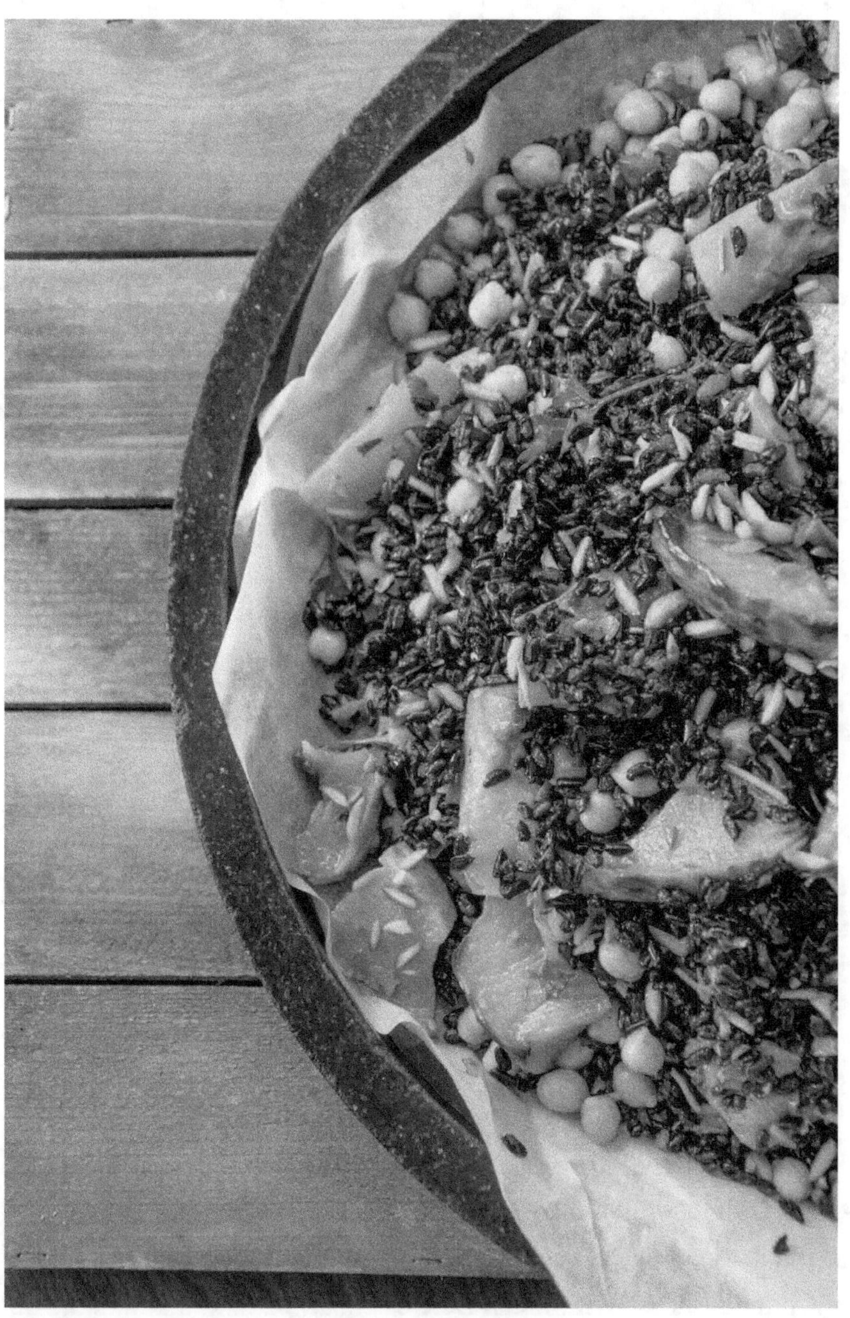

TABLE OF CONTENTS

Chapter 3: Lunch Recipes.. 42

Chapter 4: Dinner Recipes 62

Chapter 5: Snacks and Appetizers 83

INTRODUCTION

For those managing diabetes, the world of food can sometimes feel like a minefield. But what if there was a dietary approach that could be both delicious and supportive of your health goals? Enter vegetarianism! Let's delve into the world of diabetes and vegetarianism, exploring the benefits, essential nutrients, and tips for creating a vibrant and satisfying meal plan.

Understanding Diabetes and Vegetarianism:

- **Diabetes**: This chronic condition affects how your body regulates blood sugar (glucose). There are two main types: Type 1 (body doesn't produce insulin) and Type 2 (body resists insulin or doesn't produce enough).
- **Vegetarianism**: This dietary pattern excludes meat, poultry, and fish. There are various levels of vegetarianism: Lacto-ovo (includes dairy and eggs), lacto (dairy only), ovo (eggs only), and vegan (no animal products).

Benefits of a Diabetic Vegetarian Diet:

- **Weight Management**: Vegetarian diets tend to be lower in calories and fat, aiding in weight control, a crucial factor in managing diabetes.
- **Blood Sugar Control**: Plant-based foods are often rich in fiber, which helps regulate blood sugar spikes.
- **Reduced Heart Disease Risk**: Vegetarian diets are generally lower in saturated fat and cholesterol, promoting heart health, often compromised in diabetes.
- **Increased Nutrient Intake**: Plant-based diets are naturally packed with vitamins, minerals, and antioxidants, essential for overall well-being.

Essential Nutrients for Diabetic Vegetarians:

- **Protein**: Beans, lentils, tofu, tempeh, nuts, and seeds are excellent sources. Aim for variety to ensure a complete amino acid profile.
- **Healthy Fats**: Include nuts, seeds, avocados, and olive oil for satiety and nutrient absorption.
- **Iron**: Leafy greens, fortified cereals, lentils, and tofu are good options. Pair iron-rich foods with vitamin C sources (citrus fruits, peppers) to enhance absorption.

- **Calcium**: Dairy products (lacto vegetarians) or fortified plant-based milks, dark leafy greens, tofu with calcium sulfate.
- **Vitamin B12**: Fortified cereals, nutritional yeast (vegans). Consult your doctor for supplementation if needed.

Tips for Meal Planning and Preparation:

- Plan Your Week: Dedicate time to create a balanced meal plan incorporating all essential nutrients.
- Stock Up on Staples: Keep your pantry and refrigerator well-stocked with beans, lentils, whole grains, vegetables, and healthy fats.
- Cook in Batches: Prepare large batches of grains, beans, or roasted vegetables for easy incorporation into meals throughout the week.
- Get Creative with Spices and Herbs: Enhance the flavor profile of your meals with a variety of spices and herbs, reducing reliance on salt and added sugars.
- Embrace Vegetarian Staples: Explore delicious vegetarian recipes like lentil soups, veggie stir-fries, bean burritos, tofu scrambles, and whole-wheat pasta dishes.
- Read Food Labels: Be mindful of hidden sugars and saturated fats, especially in processed vegetarian foods.

By embracing a well-planned vegetarian diet, you can embark on a delicious journey that supports your diabetes management and overall well-being. Remember, consulting a registered dietitian familiar with both diabetes and vegetarianism can provide personalized guidance for your specific needs. So, explore the vibrant world of plant-based foods and discover a new path to health and culinary delight!

Chapter 1: 30 Day Meal Plan

Week 1:

Day 1:

- Breakfast: Avocado and Spinach Smoothie Bowl
- Lunch: Chickpea and Avocado Salad
- Dinner: Vegetable Stir-Fry with Tofu
- Snack: Hummus and Veggie Sticks
- Dessert: Chia Seed Pudding with Fresh Berries

Day 2:

- Breakfast: Quinoa and Berry Breakfast Bowl
- Lunch: Lentil Soup with Spinach
- Dinner: Stuffed Bell Peppers with Quinoa
- Snack: Roasted Chickpeas
- Dessert: Almond Flour Chocolate Chip Cookies

Day 3:

- Breakfast: Chia Seed Pudding with Almond Milk
- Lunch: Grilled Vegetable and Hummus Wrap
- Dinner: Eggplant Parmesan
- Snack: Stuffed Mini Bell Peppers
- Dessert: Greek Yogurt Parfait with Mixed Berries

Day 4:

- Breakfast: Scrambled Tofu with Vegetables
- Lunch: Quinoa and Black Bean Salad
- Dinner: Spinach and Ricotta Stuffed Shells
- Snack: Edamame with Sea Salt
- Dessert: Baked Apples with Cinnamon

Day 5:

- Breakfast: Greek Yogurt with Nuts and Seeds
- Lunch: Cauliflower Rice Stir-Fry
- Dinner: Zucchini Noodles with Pesto
- Snack: Spicy Avocado Dip with Whole Grain Crackers
- Dessert: Sugar-Free Chocolate Avocado Mousse

Day 6:

- Breakfast: Oatmeal with Cinnamon and Walnuts
- Lunch: Tomato Basil Soup
- Dinner: Cauliflower Pizza with Veggie Toppings
- Snack: Cucumber and Tomato Salad
- Dessert: Carrot Cake Energy Balls

Day 7:

- Breakfast: Vegetable Frittata
- Lunch: Spinach and Feta Stuffed Peppers

- Dinner: Lentil and Sweet Potato Curry

- Snack: Greek Yogurt with Honey and Nuts

- Dessert: Coconut Macaroons

Week 2:

Day 8:

- Breakfast: Green Smoothie with Kale and Cucumber

- Lunch: Roasted Beet and Goat Cheese Salad

- Dinner: Portobello Mushroom Burgers

- Snack: Baked Zucchini Chips

- Dessert: Strawberry and Basil Sorbet

Day 9:

- Breakfast: Berry and Almond Overnight Oats

- Lunch: Broccoli and Cheddar Soup

- Dinner: Butternut Squash Risotto

- Snack: Cauliflower Buffalo Bites

- Dessert: Dark Chocolate and Nut Clusters

Day 10:

- Breakfast: Buckwheat Pancakes with Fresh Fruit

- Lunch: Thai Peanut Noodle Salad

- Dinner: Spaghetti Squash with Marinara Sauce

- Snack: Guacamole with Jicama Sticks
- Dessert: Vegan Blueberry Muffins

Day 11:

- Breakfast: Cottage Cheese with Fresh Berries
- Lunch: Eggplant and Zucchini Ratatouille
- Dinner: Greek-Style Stuffed Tomatoes
- Snack: Cottage Cheese with Pineapple
- Dessert: Matcha Green Tea Ice Cream

Day 12:

- Breakfast: Spinach and Mushroom Breakfast Burrito
- Lunch: Spicy Chickpea and Carrot Salad
- Dinner: Mixed Vegetable Paella
- Snack: Vegan Sushi Rolls
- Dessert: Lemon Chia Seed Muffins

Day 13:

- Breakfast: Peanut Butter Banana Toast on Whole Grain Bread
- Lunch: Caprese Salad with Balsamic Glaze
- Dinner: Vegan Shepherd's Pie
- Snack: Spinach and Artichoke Dip
- Dessert: Banana Nice Cream

Day 14:

- Breakfast: Apple Cinnamon Quinoa
- Lunch: Tofu and Vegetable Skewers
- Dinner: Chickpea and Spinach Stew
- Snack: Caprese Skewers
- Dessert: Pumpkin Pie Bites

Week 3:

Day 15:

- Breakfast: Avocado and Spinach Smoothie Bowl
- Lunch: Chickpea and Avocado Salad
- Dinner: Vegetable Stir-Fry with Tofu
- Snack: Hummus and Veggie Sticks
- Dessert: Chia Seed Pudding with Fresh Berries

Day 16:

- Breakfast: Quinoa and Berry Breakfast Bowl
- Lunch: Lentil Soup with Spinach
- Dinner: Stuffed Bell Peppers with Quinoa
- Snack: Roasted Chickpeas
- Dessert: Almond Flour Chocolate Chip Cookies

Day 17:

- Breakfast: Chia Seed Pudding with Almond Milk
- Lunch: Grilled Vegetable and Hummus Wrap
- Dinner: Eggplant Parmesan
- Snack: Stuffed Mini Bell Peppers
- Dessert: Greek Yogurt Parfait with Mixed Berries

Day 18:

- Breakfast: Scrambled Tofu with Vegetables
- Lunch: Quinoa and Black Bean Salad
- Dinner: Spinach and Ricotta Stuffed Shells
- Snack: Edamame with Sea Salt
- Dessert: Baked Apples with Cinnamon

Day 19:

- Breakfast: Greek Yogurt with Nuts and Seeds
- Lunch: Cauliflower Rice Stir-Fry
- Dinner: Zucchini Noodles with Pesto
- Snack: Spicy Avocado Dip with Whole Grain Crackers
- Dessert: Sugar-Free Chocolate Avocado Mousse

Day 20:

- Breakfast: Oatmeal with Cinnamon and Walnuts
- Lunch: Tomato Basil Soup

- Dinner: Cauliflower Pizza with Veggie Toppings
- Snack: Cucumber and Tomato Salad
- Dessert: Carrot Cake Energy Balls

Day 21:

- Breakfast: Vegetable Frittata
- Lunch: Spinach and Feta Stuffed Peppers
- Dinner: Lentil and Sweet Potato Curry
- Snack: Greek Yogurt with Honey and Nuts
- Dessert: Coconut Macaroons

Week 4:

Day 22:

- Breakfast: Berry and Almond Overnight Oats
- Lunch: Broccoli and Cheddar Soup
- Dinner: Butternut Squash Risotto
- Snack: Cauliflower Buffalo Bites
- Dessert: Dark Chocolate and Nut Clusters

Day 23:

- Breakfast: Buckwheat Pancakes with Fresh Fruit
- Lunch: Thai Peanut Noodle Salad
- Dinner: Spaghetti Squash with Marinara Sauce

- Snack: Guacamole with Jicama Sticks
- Dessert: Vegan Blueberry Muffins

Day 24:

- Breakfast: Cottage Cheese with Fresh Berries
- Lunch: Eggplant and Zucchini Ratatouille
- Dinner: Greek-Style Stuffed Tomatoes
- Snack: Cottage Cheese with Pineapple
- Dessert: Matcha Green Tea Ice Cream

Day 25:

- Breakfast: Spinach and Mushroom Breakfast Burrito
- Lunch: Spicy Chickpea and Carrot Salad
- Dinner: Mixed Vegetable Paella
- Snack: Vegan Sushi Rolls
- Dessert: Lemon Chia Seed Muffins

Day 26:

- Breakfast: Peanut Butter Banana Toast on Whole Grain Bread
- Lunch: Caprese Salad with Balsamic Glaze
- Dinner: Vegan Shepherd's Pie
- Snack: Spinach and Artichoke Dip
- Dessert: Banana Nice Cream

Day 27:

- Breakfast: Apple Cinnamon Quinoa
- Lunch: Tofu and Vegetable Skewers
- Dinner: Chickpea and Spinach Stew
- Snack: Caprese Skewers
- Dessert: Pumpkin Pie Bites

Day 28:

- Breakfast: Avocado and Spinach Smoothie Bowl
- Lunch: Chickpea and Avocado Salad
- Dinner: Vegetable Stir-Fry with Tofu
- Snack: Hummus and Veggie Sticks
- Dessert: Chia Seed Pudding with Fresh Berries

Day 29:

- Breakfast: Quinoa and Berry Breakfast Bowl
- Lunch: Lentil Soup with Spinach
- Dinner: Stuffed Bell Peppers with Quinoa
- Snack: Roasted Chickpeas
- Dessert: Almond Flour Chocolate Chip Cookies

Day 30:

- Breakfast: Chia Seed Pudding with Almond Milk
- Lunch: Grilled Vegetable and Hummus Wrap

- Dinner: Eggplant Parmesan
- Snack: Stuffed Mini Bell Peppers
- Dessert: Greek Yogurt Parfait with Mixed Berries

Chapter 2: Breakfast Recipes

These breakfast recipes are not only delicious but also packed with essential nutrients to fuel your day. From smoothie bowls to hearty burritos, there's something here to satisfy every craving.

Avocado and Spinach Smoothie Bowl

Ingredients:

- 1 ripe avocado
- 1 cup spinach leaves
- 1 banana
- 1/2 cup almond milk
- 1 tablespoon honey
- Toppings of choice: sliced strawberries, granola, chia seeds

Instructions:

1. In a blender, combine avocado, spinach, banana, almond milk, and honey. Blend until smooth.
2. Pour the smoothie into a bowl and top with sliced strawberries, granola, and chia seeds.
3. Enjoy immediately.

Nutrition Information:

- Calories: 320
- Protein: 6g
- Carbohydrates: 40g
- Fat: 18g
- Fiber: 10g
- Sugar: 20g
- Portion size: 1 bowl

Quinoa and Berry Breakfast Bowl

Ingredients:

- 1/2 cup cooked quinoa
- 1/2 cup mixed berries (such as strawberries, blueberries, raspberries)
- 1 tablespoon honey
- 1/4 cup almond milk
- 1 tablespoon chopped nuts (such as almonds or walnuts)

Instructions:

1. In a bowl, combine cooked quinoa, mixed berries, honey, and almond milk.
2. Stir until well combined.
3. Top with chopped nuts.

4. Serve immediately.

Nutrition Information:

- Calories: 250
- Protein: 7g
- Carbohydrates: 40g
- Fat: 6g
- Fiber: 6g
- Sugar: 12g
- Portion size: 1 bowl

Chia Seed Pudding with Almond Milk

Ingredients:

- 1/4 cup chia seeds
- 1 cup almond milk
- 1 tablespoon maple syrup
- 1/2 teaspoon vanilla extract
- Fresh fruit for topping (such as berries or sliced banana)

Instructions:

1. In a bowl, whisk together chia seeds, almond milk, maple syrup, and vanilla extract.

2. Cover and refrigerate for at least 4 hours or overnight, until thickened.

3. Serve topped with fresh fruit.

Nutrition Information:

- Calories: 180
- Protein: 5g
- Carbohydrates: 20g
- Fat: 9g
- Fiber: 10g
- Sugar: 6g
- Portion size: 1 serving

Scrambled Tofu with Vegetables

Ingredients:

- 1 block firm tofu, crumbled
- 1 bell pepper, diced
- 1/2 onion, diced
- 1 cup spinach leaves
- 2 tablespoons nutritional yeast
- 1 teaspoon turmeric
- Salt and pepper to taste
- 1 tablespoon olive oil

Instructions:

1. Heat olive oil in a pan over medium heat.
2. Add diced bell pepper and onion, and sauté until softened.
3. Add crumbled tofu, nutritional yeast, turmeric, salt, and pepper to the pan.
4. Cook, stirring occasionally, until tofu is heated through and slightly browned.
5. Add spinach leaves and cook until wilted.
6. Serve hot.

Nutrition Information:

- Calories: 220
- Protein: 15g
- Carbohydrates: 10g
- Fat: 14g
- Fiber: 4g
- Sugar: 3g
- Portion size: 1 serving

Greek Yogurt with Nuts and Seeds

Ingredients:

- 1/2 cup Greek yogurt
- 1 tablespoon chopped nuts (such as almonds or walnuts)

- 1 tablespoon mixed seeds (such as chia seeds, flaxseeds, pumpkin seeds)
- 1 tablespoon honey or maple syrup
- Fresh fruit for topping (such as sliced strawberries or banana)

Instructions:

1. In a bowl, spoon Greek yogurt.
2. Top with chopped nuts, mixed seeds, and drizzle with honey or maple syrup.
3. Add fresh fruit on top.
4. Serve immediately.

Nutrition Information:

- Calories: 200
- Protein: 15g
- Carbohydrates: 20g
- Fat: 8g
- Fiber: 3g
- Sugar: 15g
- Portion size: 1 serving

Oatmeal with Cinnamon and Walnuts

Ingredients:

- 1/2 cup rolled oats
- 1 cup water or almond milk
- 1/2 teaspoon ground cinnamon
- 1 tablespoon chopped walnuts
- 1 tablespoon maple syrup or honey
- Fresh fruit for topping (such as sliced banana or apple)

Instructions:

1. In a small saucepan, bring water or almond milk to a boil.
2. Stir in rolled oats and reduce heat to simmer.
3. Cook for 5-7 minutes, stirring occasionally, until oats are cooked and creamy.
4. Stir in ground cinnamon and chopped walnuts.
5. Remove from heat and sweeten with maple syrup or honey.
6. Serve hot, topped with fresh fruit.

Nutrition Information:

- Calories: 280
- Protein: 7g
- Carbohydrates: 45g
- Fat: 9g
- Fiber: 7g

- Sugar: 10g
- Portion size: 1 serving

Vegetable Frittata

Ingredients:

- 4 eggs
- 1/4 cup milk or almond milk
- 1 cup chopped mixed vegetables (such as bell peppers, spinach, onions)
- Salt and pepper to taste
- 1 tablespoon olive oil

Instructions:

1. Preheat the oven to 350°F (175°C).
2. In a bowl, whisk together eggs, milk, salt, and pepper.
3. Heat olive oil in an oven-safe skillet over medium heat.
4. Add chopped vegetables to the skillet and sauté until softened.
5. Pour the egg mixture over the vegetables in the skillet.
6. Cook for 3-4 minutes, until the edges start to set.
7. Transfer the skillet to the preheated oven and bake for 10-12 minutes, until the frittata is set and golden brown.
8. Slice and serve hot.

Nutrition Information:

- Calories: 180
- Protein: 12g
- Carbohydrates: 5g
- Fat: 12g
- Fiber: 2g
- Sugar: 3g
- Portion size: 1 serving

Green Smoothie with Kale and Cucumber

Ingredients:

- 1 cup chopped kale leaves
- 1/2 cucumber, peeled and chopped
- 1 green apple, cored and chopped
- 1/2 lemon, juiced
- 1 cup coconut water or almond milk
- 1 tablespoon honey or maple syrup (optional)

Instructions:

1. In a blender, combine chopped kale, cucumber, apple, lemon juice, and coconut water or almond milk.
2. Blend until smooth.
3. Taste and add honey or maple syrup if desired for sweetness.

4. Pour into glasses and serve immediately.

Nutrition Information:

- Calories: 120
- Protein: 3g
- Carbohydrates: 25g
- Fat: 2g
- Fiber: 6g
- Sugar: 15g
- Portion size: 1 serving

Berry and Almond Overnight Oats

Ingredients:

- 1/2 cup rolled oats
- 1/2 cup almond milk
- 1/4 cup Greek yogurt
- 1/4 cup mixed berries (such as strawberries, blueberries, raspberries)
- 1 tablespoon almond butter
- 1 tablespoon honey or maple syrup
- 1 tablespoon sliced almonds

Instructions:

1. In a jar or container, combine rolled oats, almond milk, Greek yogurt, mixed berries, almond butter, and honey or maple syrup.
2. Stir until well combined.
3. Cover and refrigerate overnight.
4. In the morning, top with sliced almonds before serving.

Nutrition Information:

- Calories: 320
- Protein: 12g
- Carbohydrates: 40g
- Fat: 14g
- Fiber: 8g
- Sugar: 12g
- Portion size: 1 serving

Buckwheat Pancakes with Fresh Fruit

Ingredients:

- 1 cup buckwheat flour
- 1 tablespoon ground flaxseed
- 1 teaspoon baking powder
- 1/2 teaspoon ground cinnamon

- 1 cup almond milk
- 1 tablespoon maple syrup or honey
- Fresh fruit for topping (such as sliced bananas, berries)

Instructions:

1. In a bowl, whisk together buckwheat flour, ground flaxseed, baking powder, and ground cinnamon.
2. Stir in almond milk and maple syrup or honey until smooth batter forms.
3. Heat a non-stick skillet or griddle over medium heat.
4. Pour 1/4 cup of batter onto the skillet for each pancake.
5. Cook until bubbles form on the surface, then flip and cook until golden brown on the other side.
6. Serve hot, topped with fresh fruit.

Nutrition Information:

- Calories: 250
- Protein: 8g
- Carbohydrates: 45g
- Fat: 5g
- Fiber: 7g
- Sugar: 10g
- Portion size: 2 pancakes

Cottage Cheese with Fresh Berries

Ingredients:

- 1/2 cup low-fat cottage cheese
- 1/2 cup mixed berries (such as strawberries, blueberries, raspberries)
- 1 tablespoon honey or maple syrup
- 1 tablespoon sliced almonds or chopped walnuts

Instructions:

1. In a bowl, spoon cottage cheese.
2. Top with mixed berries and drizzle with honey or maple syrup.
3. Sprinkle with sliced almonds or chopped walnuts.
4. Serve immediately.

Nutrition Information:

- Calories: 200
- Protein: 15g
- Carbohydrates: 20g
- Fat: 8g
- Fiber: 5g
- Sugar: 12g
- Portion size: 1 serving

Spinach and Mushroom Breakfast Burrito

Ingredients:

- 2 large whole grain tortillas
- 1 cup spinach leaves
- 1 cup sliced mushrooms
- 4 eggs, beaten
- 1/4 cup shredded cheese (optional)
- Salt and pepper to taste
- Salsa or hot sauce for serving

Instructions:

1. Heat a non-stick skillet over medium heat.
2. Add spinach and mushrooms to the skillet and cook until wilted and tender.
3. Pour beaten eggs over the spinach and mushrooms in the skillet.
4. Cook, stirring occasionally, until the eggs are scrambled and cooked through.
5. Divide the egg mixture between the two tortillas.
6. Sprinkle shredded cheese on top if desired.
7. Roll up the tortillas to form burritos.
8. Serve with salsa or hot sauce on the side.

Nutrition Information:

- Calories: 320
- Protein: 18g
- Carbohydrates: 25g
- Fat: 15g
- Fiber: 5g
- Sugar: 3g
- Portion size: 1 burrito

Peanut Butter Banana Toast on Whole Grain Bread

Ingredients:

- 2 slices whole grain bread, toasted
- 2 tablespoons peanut butter
- 1 banana, sliced
- 1 tablespoon honey or maple syrup (optional)
- Pinch of cinnamon (optional)

Instructions:

1. Spread peanut butter evenly on toasted whole grain bread slices.
2. Arrange sliced banana on top of the peanut butter.

3. Drizzle with honey or maple syrup if desired, and sprinkle with a pinch of cinnamon.

4. Serve immediately.

Nutrition Information:

- Calories: 350
- Protein: 10g
- Carbohydrates: 40g
- Fat: 18g
- Fiber: 7g
- Sugar: 15g
- Portion size: 1 serving

Apple Cinnamon Quinoa

Ingredients:

- 1/2 cup quinoa
- 1 cup water or almond milk
- 1 apple, diced
- 1 tablespoon maple syrup or honey
- 1/2 teaspoon ground cinnamon
- 1 tablespoon chopped nuts (such as almonds or walnuts)

Instructions:

1. Rinse quinoa under cold water.
2. In a saucepan, combine quinoa and water or almond milk.
3. Bring to a boil, then reduce heat to low, cover, and simmer for 15 minutes, or until quinoa is cooked and liquid is absorbed.
4. Stir in diced apple, maple syrup or honey, and ground cinnamon.
5. Cook for an additional 2-3 minutes until apple is softened.
6. Remove from heat and top with chopped nuts.
7. Serve hot.

Nutrition Information:

- Calories: 280
- Protein: 8g
- Carbohydrates: 45g
- Fat: 8g
- Fiber: 7g
- Sugar: 15g
- Portion size: 1 serving

Spiced Lentil and Veggie Breakfast Hash

Ingredients:

- 1 cup cooked lentils
- 1 cup diced mixed vegetables (such as bell peppers, onions, zucchini)
- 1/2 teaspoon ground cumin
- 1/2 teaspoon paprika
- Salt and pepper to taste
- 1 tablespoon olive oil
- 2 eggs (optional)

Instructions:

1. Heat olive oil in a skillet over medium heat.
2. Add diced mixed vegetables to the skillet and sauté until softened.
3. Stir in cooked lentils, ground cumin, paprika, salt, and pepper.
4. Cook for an additional 3-4 minutes until heated through and flavors are combined.
5. If desired, make two wells in the hash and crack an egg into each well.
6. Cover and cook until eggs are cooked to your liking.
7. Serve hot.

Nutrition Information:

- Calories: 320
- Protein: 18g
- Carbohydrates: 30g
- Fat: 15g
- Fiber: 10g
- Sugar: 5g
- Portion size: 1 serving

Chapter 3: Lunch Recipes

Lunch not only provides energy to sustain you throughout the day but also offers an opportunity to incorporate essential nutrients into your diet. These recipes are designed to be flavorful, satisfying, and packed with wholesome ingredients to fuel your body and mind.

Chickpea and Avocado Salad

Ingredients:

- 1 can chickpeas, drained and rinsed
- 1 ripe avocado, diced
- 1 cup cherry tomatoes, halved
- 1/4 cup red onion, finely chopped
- 2 tablespoons fresh cilantro, chopped
- 1 tablespoon olive oil
- 1 tablespoon lemon juice
- Salt and pepper to taste

Instructions:

1. In a large bowl, combine chickpeas, avocado, cherry tomatoes, red onion, and cilantro.
2. Drizzle olive oil and lemon juice over the salad.
3. Season with salt and pepper, then toss gently to coat.

4. Serve chilled.

Nutrition Information (per serving):

- Calories: 280
- Protein: 9g
- Carbohydrates: 23g
- Fat: 17g
- Fiber: 9g
- Sugar: 3g
- Portion size: 1 cup

Lentil Soup with Spinach

Ingredients:

- 1 cup green lentils, rinsed
- 4 cups vegetable broth
- 2 cups spinach leaves
- 1 onion, diced
- 2 cloves garlic, minced
- 1 carrot, diced
- 1 celery stalk, diced
- 1 teaspoon cumin
- Salt and pepper to taste

Instructions:

1. In a large pot, sauté onion, garlic, carrot, and celery until softened.
2. Add lentils, vegetable broth, and cumin to the pot. Bring to a boil, then reduce heat and simmer for 20-25 minutes, until lentils are tender.
3. Stir in spinach leaves and cook until wilted.
4. Season with salt and pepper before serving.

Nutrition Information (per serving):

- Calories: 220
- Protein: 13g
- Carbohydrates: 38g
- Fat: 1g
- Fiber: 15g
- Sugar: 4g
- Portion size: 1.5 cups

Grilled Vegetable and Hummus Wrap

Ingredients:

- 1 large whole wheat tortilla
- 1/4 cup hummus

- 1/2 cup mixed grilled vegetables (such as bell peppers, zucchini, and eggplant)
- Handful of baby spinach leaves
- 1 tablespoon chopped fresh herbs (such as parsley or cilantro)

Instructions:

1. Spread hummus evenly over the whole wheat tortilla.
2. Arrange the grilled vegetables and baby spinach leaves on top of the hummus.
3. Sprinkle with chopped fresh herbs.
4. Roll up the tortilla tightly, slice in half if desired, and serve.

Nutrition Information (per serving):

- Calories: 280
- Protein: 8g
- Carbohydrates: 36g
- Fat: 12g
- Fiber: 8g
- Sugar: 3g
- Portion size: 1 wrap

Quinoa and Black Bean Salad

Ingredients:

- 1 cup cooked quinoa
- 1 can black beans, drained and rinsed
- 1 cup cherry tomatoes, halved
- 1/4 cup red onion, finely chopped
- 1/4 cup fresh cilantro, chopped
- 2 tablespoons lime juice
- 1 tablespoon olive oil
- Salt and pepper to taste

Instructions:

1. In a large bowl, combine cooked quinoa, black beans, cherry tomatoes, red onion, and cilantro.
2. Drizzle lime juice and olive oil over the salad.
3. Season with salt and pepper, then toss gently to combine.
4. Serve chilled or at room temperature.

Nutrition Information (per serving):

- Calories: 290
- Protein: 11g
- Carbohydrates: 48g
- Fat: 6g
- Fiber: 12g

- Sugar: 2g
- Portion size: 1 cup

Cauliflower Rice Stir-Fry

Ingredients:

- 1 head cauliflower, grated into rice-like texture
- 1 cup mixed vegetables (such as bell peppers, broccoli, and carrots)
- 1/4 cup soy sauce (or tamari for gluten-free option)
- 2 cloves garlic, minced
- 1 tablespoon sesame oil
- 2 green onions, thinly sliced

Instructions:

1. In a large skillet or wok, heat sesame oil over medium heat. Add minced garlic and cook until fragrant.
2. Add grated cauliflower rice and mixed vegetables to the skillet. Stir-fry for 5-7 minutes until vegetables are tender.
3. Pour soy sauce over the cauliflower rice mixture and continue to cook for another 2-3 minutes.
4. Garnish with sliced green onions before serving.

Nutrition Information (per serving):

- Calories: 150

- Protein: 6g

- Carbohydrates: 20g

- Fat: 7g

- Fiber: 8g

- Sugar: 6g

- Portion size: 1.5 cups

Tomato Basil Soup

Ingredients:

- 4 large tomatoes, diced

- 1 onion, chopped

- 2 cloves garlic, minced

- 1 tablespoon olive oil

- 2 cups vegetable broth

- 1/4 cup fresh basil leaves, chopped

- Salt and pepper to taste

Instructions:

1. In a large pot, heat olive oil over medium heat. Add chopped onion and garlic, sauté until softened.

2. Add diced tomatoes to the pot and cook until they start to break down.

3. Pour in vegetable broth and bring to a simmer. Let it cook for 15-20 minutes.

4. Stir in fresh basil leaves and season with salt and pepper.

5. Blend the soup until smooth using an immersion blender or transfer to a blender in batches.

6. Serve hot, garnished with additional fresh basil leaves if desired.

Nutrition Information (per serving):

- Calories: 120
- Protein: 3g
- Carbohydrates: 16g
- Fat: 6g
- Fiber: 4g
- Sugar: 8g
- Portion size: 1 cup

Spinach and Feta Stuffed Peppers

Ingredients:

- 4 bell peppers, halved and seeds removed
- 2 cups cooked quinoa

- 1 cup baby spinach, chopped
- 1/2 cup crumbled feta cheese
- 1/4 cup pine nuts
- 1 teaspoon dried oregano
- Salt and pepper to taste

Instructions:

1. Preheat the oven to 375°F (190°C). Place halved bell peppers in a baking dish.
2. In a mixing bowl, combine cooked quinoa, chopped baby spinach, crumbled feta cheese, pine nuts, dried oregano, salt, and pepper.
3. Spoon the quinoa mixture evenly into each bell pepper half.
4. Cover the baking dish with aluminum foil and bake for 25-30 minutes, or until peppers are tender.
5. Serve hot as a delicious and nutritious lunch option.

Nutrition Information (per serving):

- Calories: 240
- Protein: 9g
- Carbohydrates: 30g
- Fat: 10g
- Fiber: 6g
- Sugar: 7g

- Portion size: 1 stuffed pepper half

Roasted Beet and Goat Cheese Salad

Ingredients:

- 4 medium beets, peeled and diced
- 2 tablespoons olive oil
- 4 cups mixed greens
- 1/2 cup crumbled goat cheese
- 1/4 cup walnuts, chopped
- 2 tablespoons balsamic vinegar
- Salt and pepper to taste

Instructions:

1. Preheat the oven to 400°F (200°C). Place diced beets on a baking sheet and toss with olive oil, salt, and pepper.
2. Roast in the oven for 25-30 minutes, or until beets are tender and slightly caramelized.
3. In a large bowl, combine mixed greens, roasted beets, crumbled goat cheese, and chopped walnuts.
4. Drizzle balsamic vinegar over the salad and toss gently to coat.
5. Serve immediately as a vibrant and flavorful lunch option.

Nutrition Information (per serving):

- Calories: 280
- Protein: 9g
- Carbohydrates: 20g
- Fat: 18g
- Fiber: 6g
- Sugar: 12g
- Portion size: 2 cups

Broccoli and Cheddar Soup

Ingredients:

- 2 cups broccoli florets
- 1 onion, diced
- 2 cloves garlic, minced
- 2 cups vegetable broth
- 1 cup milk (or dairy-free alternative)
- 1 cup shredded cheddar cheese (or dairy-free alternative)
- Salt and pepper to taste

Instructions:

1. In a large pot, sauté diced onion and minced garlic until softened.

2. Add broccoli florets and vegetable broth to the pot. Bring to a boil, then reduce heat and simmer for 10-15 minutes until broccoli is tender.

3. Use an immersion blender to blend the soup until smooth. Alternatively, transfer the soup to a blender and blend in batches.

4. Stir in milk and shredded cheddar cheese until cheese is melted and incorporated.

5. Season with salt and pepper to taste.

6. Serve hot with a sprinkle of shredded cheese on top, if desired.

Nutrition Information (per serving):

- Calories: 220
- Protein: 12g
- Carbohydrates: 14g
- Fat: 14g
- Fiber: 3g
- Sugar: 6g
- Portion size: 1.5 cups

Thai Peanut Noodle Salad

Ingredients:

- 8 oz whole wheat spaghetti noodles (or rice noodles for gluten-free option)
- 1/2 cup peanut butter
- 1/4 cup soy sauce (or tamari for gluten-free option)
- 2 tablespoons rice vinegar
- 1 tablespoon sesame oil
- 1 tablespoon honey (or maple syrup for vegan option)
- 1 teaspoon grated ginger
- 2 cloves garlic, minced
- 1 bell pepper, thinly sliced
- 1 carrot, julienned
- 1/4 cup chopped peanuts
- Fresh cilantro for garnish

Instructions:

1. Cook spaghetti noodles according to package instructions. Drain and rinse under cold water.
2. In a small bowl, whisk together peanut butter, soy sauce, rice vinegar, sesame oil, honey, grated ginger, and minced garlic to make the dressing.
3. In a large bowl, combine cooked spaghetti noodles, sliced bell pepper, julienned carrot, and chopped peanuts.

4. Pour the dressing over the noodle mixture and toss until evenly coated.

5. Garnish with fresh cilantro before serving.

6. Serve chilled or at room temperature.

Nutrition Information (per serving):

- Calories: 380
- Protein: 15g
- Carbohydrates: 48g
- Fat: 16g
- Fiber: 7g
- Sugar: 7g
- Portion size: 2 cups

Eggplant and Zucchini Ratatouille

Ingredients:

- 1 eggplant, diced
- 2 zucchinis, diced
- 1 onion, diced
- 2 cloves garlic, minced
- 1 can diced tomatoes
- 1 teaspoon dried thyme
- 1 teaspoon dried oregano

- Salt and pepper to taste
- Fresh basil for garnish

Instructions:

1. In a large skillet, heat olive oil over medium heat. Add diced onion and minced garlic, sauté until softened.
2. Add diced eggplant and zucchinis to the skillet, cook until vegetables are slightly tender.
3. Stir in diced tomatoes, dried thyme, and dried oregano. Season with salt and pepper to taste.
4. Cover and let simmer for 15-20 minutes, stirring occasionally, until vegetables are fully cooked.
5. Garnish with fresh basil before serving.
6. Serve hot as a satisfying and flavorful lunch option.

Nutrition Information (per serving):

- Calories: 180
- Protein: 5g
- Carbohydrates: 30g
- Fat: 7g
- Fiber: 10g
- Sugar: 14g
- Portion size: 1.5 cups

Spicy Chickpea and Carrot Salad

Ingredients:

- 1 can chickpeas, drained and rinsed
- 2 carrots, grated
- 1/4 cup chopped fresh cilantro
- 2 tablespoons olive oil
- 1 tablespoon lemon juice
- 1 teaspoon ground cumin
- 1/2 teaspoon chili powder
- Salt and pepper to taste

Instructions:

1. In a large bowl, combine chickpeas, grated carrots, and chopped cilantro.
2. In a small bowl, whisk together olive oil, lemon juice, ground cumin, chili powder, salt, and pepper to make the dressing.
3. Pour the dressing over the chickpea and carrot mixture, toss until evenly coated.
4. Serve chilled or at room temperature.

Nutrition Information (per serving):

- Calories: 220
- Protein: 6g

- Carbohydrates: 27g
- Fat: 10g
- Fiber: 7g
- Sugar: 6g
- Portion size: 1 cup

Caprese Salad with Balsamic Glaze

Ingredients:

- 2 large tomatoes, sliced
- 1 ball fresh mozzarella cheese, sliced
- Handful of fresh basil leaves
- 2 tablespoons balsamic glaze
- Salt and pepper to taste

Instructions:

1. Arrange sliced tomatoes and fresh mozzarella cheese on a serving platter.
2. Tuck fresh basil leaves in between the tomato and mozzarella slices.
3. Drizzle balsamic glaze over the salad.
4. Season with salt and pepper to taste.
5. Serve immediately as a light and refreshing lunch option.

Nutrition Information (per serving):

- Calories: 250
- Protein: 14g
- Carbohydrates: 10g
- Fat: 18g
- Fiber: 2g
- Sugar: 6g
- Portion size: 1 plate

Tofu and Vegetable Skewers

Ingredients:

- 1 block extra-firm tofu, cubed
- 1 bell pepper, cut into chunks
- 1 zucchini, sliced
- 1 red onion, cut into chunks
- 1/4 cup soy sauce (or tamari for gluten-free option)
- 2 tablespoons maple syrup
- 1 tablespoon sesame oil
- 2 cloves garlic, minced

Instructions:

1. In a small bowl, whisk together soy sauce, maple syrup, sesame oil, and minced garlic to make the marinade.

2. Thread tofu cubes, bell pepper chunks, zucchini slices, and red onion chunks onto skewers.

3. Place the skewers in a shallow dish and pour the marinade over them. Let them marinate for at least 30 minutes.

4. Preheat the grill or grill pan over medium-high heat. Grill the skewers for 8-10 minutes, turning occasionally, until vegetables are tender and tofu is lightly charred.

5. Serve hot as a protein-packed lunch option.

Nutrition Information (per serving):

- Calories: 280
- Protein: 18g
- Carbohydrates: 24g
- Fat: 12g
- Fiber: 6g
- Sugar: 12g
- Portion size: 2 skewers

Mediterranean Farro Salad

Ingredients:

- 1 cup cooked farro
- 1 cup cherry tomatoes, halved
- 1 cucumber, diced

- 1/4 cup Kalamata olives, pitted and halved
- 1/4 cup crumbled feta cheese
- 2 tablespoons chopped fresh parsley
- 2 tablespoons lemon juice
- 1 tablespoon olive oil
- Salt and pepper to taste

Instructions:

1. In a large bowl, combine cooked farro, halved cherry tomatoes, diced cucumber, halved Kalamata olives, crumbled feta cheese, and chopped fresh parsley.
2. Drizzle lemon juice and olive oil over the salad.
3. Season with salt and pepper to taste.
4. Toss gently to combine.
5. Serve chilled or at room temperature.

Nutrition Information (per serving):

- Calories: 270
- Protein: 8g
- Carbohydrates: 38g
- Fat: 10g
- Fiber: 8g
- Sugar: 4g
- Portion size: 1 cup

Chapter 4: Dinner Recipes

In this Chapter, you'll find a delightful array of dinner recipes perfect for satisfying your taste buds while nourishing your body. From hearty casseroles to flavorful stir-fries, these recipes are designed to make your evenings both delicious and nutritious.

Vegetable Stir-Fry with Tofu

Ingredients:

- Tofu
- Mixed vegetables (bell peppers, broccoli, carrots, snap peas)
- Soy sauce
- Garlic
- Ginger
- Olive oil
- Sesame seeds

Instructions:

1. Press tofu to remove excess moisture, then cut into cubes.
2. Heat olive oil in a pan and sauté garlic and ginger until fragrant.
3. Add tofu and cook until golden brown.
4. Add mixed vegetables and stir-fry until tender.

5. Season with soy sauce and sprinkle with sesame seeds before serving.

Nutrition Information:

- Calories: 250
- Protein: 15g
- Carbohydrates: 20g
- Fat: 12g
- Fiber: 8g
- Sugar: 6g
- Portion size: 1 serving

Stuffed Bell Peppers with Quinoa

Ingredients:

- Bell peppers
- Quinoa
- Black beans
- Corn
- Onion
- Garlic
- Tomato sauce
- Mexican seasoning
- Cheese (optional)

Instructions:

1. Cook quinoa according to package instructions.
2. Sauté onion and garlic, then mix with cooked quinoa, black beans, corn, and tomato sauce.
3. Cut tops off bell peppers and remove seeds.
4. Stuff peppers with quinoa mixture and sprinkle with cheese if desired.
5. Bake until peppers are tender and filling is heated through.

Nutrition Information:

- Calories: 300
- Protein: 12g
- Carbohydrates: 40g
- Fat: 8g
- Fiber: 10g
- Sugar: 8g
- Portion size: 1 stuffed pepper

Eggplant Parmesan

Ingredients:

- Eggplant
- Marinara sauce
- Mozzarella cheese

- Parmesan cheese
- Bread crumbs
- Italian seasoning

Instructions:

1. Slice eggplant into rounds, then coat in bread crumbs mixed with Italian seasoning.
2. Bake eggplant until golden brown and crispy.
3. Layer eggplant slices with marinara sauce and cheeses in a baking dish.
4. Bake until cheese is melted and bubbly.
5. Serve hot with a side of spaghetti or salad.

Nutrition Information:

- Calories: 280
- Protein: 15g
- Carbohydrates: 25g
- Fat: 15g
- Fiber: 8g
- Sugar: 10g
- Portion size: 1 serving

Spinach and Ricotta Stuffed Shells

Ingredients:

- Jumbo pasta shells
- Ricotta cheese
- Spinach
- Garlic
- Mozzarella cheese
- Parmesan cheese
- Marinara sauce

Instructions:

1. Cook pasta shells according to package instructions.
2. Sauté garlic and spinach until wilted, then mix with ricotta cheese.
3. Stuff cooked shells with spinach and ricotta mixture.
4. Arrange stuffed shells in a baking dish, top with marinara sauce and cheeses.
5. Bake until cheese is melted and bubbly.

Nutrition Information:

- Calories: 320
- Protein: 18g
- Carbohydrates: 30g
- Fat: 15g

- Fiber: 5g

- Sugar: 8g

- Portion size: 3 shells

Zucchini Noodles with Pesto

Ingredients:

- Zucchini

- Basil

- Pine nuts

- Garlic

- Olive oil

- Parmesan cheese

- Lemon juice

Instructions:

1. Spiralize zucchini into noodles.

2. Blend basil, pine nuts, garlic, olive oil, and Parmesan cheese to make pesto.

3. Toss zucchini noodles with pesto until well coated.

4. Sauté noodles until heated through.

5. Serve with a squeeze of lemon juice and additional Parmesan cheese if desired.

Nutrition Information:

- Calories: 200
- Protein: 8g
- Carbohydrates: 15g
- Fat: 15g
- Fiber: 5g
- Sugar: 4g
- Portion size: 1 serving

Cauliflower Pizza with Veggie Toppings

Ingredients:

- Cauliflower
- Eggs
- Mozzarella cheese
- Italian seasoning
- Tomato sauce
- Bell peppers
- Mushrooms
- Red onion
- Olives
- Spinach

Instructions:

1. Rice cauliflower and microwave until tender, then squeeze out excess moisture.
2. Mix cauliflower with eggs, mozzarella cheese, and Italian seasoning to form a dough.
3. Press dough onto a baking sheet and bake until golden brown.
4. Top crust with tomato sauce and your choice of vegetables.
5. Bake pizza until toppings are heated through and cheese is melted.

Nutrition Information:

- Calories: 220
- Protein: 10g
- Carbohydrates: 20g
- Fat: 10g
- Fiber: 8g
- Sugar: 6g
- Portion size: 1 slice

Lentil and Sweet Potato Curry

Ingredients:

- Lentils

- Sweet potatoes
- Onion
- Garlic
- Ginger
- Coconut milk
- Curry powder
- Vegetable broth
- Spinach

Instructions:

1. Sauté onion, garlic, and ginger until fragrant.
2. Add lentils, diced sweet potatoes, curry powder, coconut milk, and vegetable broth.
3. Simmer until lentils and sweet potatoes are tender.
4. Stir in spinach until wilted.
5. Serve hot over rice or quinoa.

Nutrition Information:

- Calories: 280
- Protein: 12g
- Carbohydrates: 30g
- Fat: 10g
- Fiber: 12g
- Sugar: 8g

- Portion size: 1 serving

Portobello Mushroom Burgers

Ingredients:

- Portobello mushrooms
- Buns (whole wheat or gluten-free)
- Red onion
- Tomato
- Lettuce
- Avocado
- Balsamic vinegar
- Olive oil
- Garlic powder
- Salt and pepper

Instructions:

1. Marinate portobello mushrooms in a mixture of balsamic vinegar, olive oil, garlic powder, salt, and pepper.
2. Grill mushrooms until tender, about 5-7 minutes per side.
3. Toast buns on the grill.
4. Assemble burgers with grilled mushrooms, sliced tomato, onion, lettuce, and avocado.
5. Serve hot with your favorite condiments.

Nutrition Information:

- Calories: 260
- Protein: 8g
- Carbohydrates: 30g
- Fat: 12g
- Fiber: 10g
- Sugar: 6g
- Portion size: 1 burger

Butternut Squash Risotto

Ingredients:

- Arborio rice
- Butternut squash
- Onion
- Garlic
- Vegetable broth
- Parmesan cheese
- White wine (optional)
- Sage
- Olive oil

Instructions:

1. Sauté onion and garlic in olive oil until translucent.

2. Add Arborio rice and cook until lightly toasted.

3. Stir in diced butternut squash and chopped sage.

4. Gradually add vegetable broth, stirring frequently, until rice is creamy and tender.

5. Stir in Parmesan cheese and season with salt and pepper to taste.

Nutrition Information:

- Calories: 300
- Protein: 8g
- Carbohydrates: 40g
- Fat: 10g
- Fiber: 6g
- Sugar: 6g
- Portion size: 1 serving

Spaghetti Squash with Marinara Sauce

Ingredients:

- Spaghetti squash
- Marinara sauce (store-bought or homemade)
- Olive oil
- Garlic
- Italian seasoning

- Salt and pepper
- Fresh basil (optional)
- Parmesan cheese (optional)

Instructions:

1. Preheat oven to 400°F (200°C).
2. Cut spaghetti squash in half lengthwise and scoop out seeds.
3. Drizzle cut sides with olive oil and sprinkle with minced garlic, Italian seasoning, salt, and pepper.
4. Place squash halves cut-side down on a baking sheet and roast for 30-40 minutes, or until tender.
5. Use a fork to scrape out the strands of squash into a bowl.
6. Heat marinara sauce in a saucepan until heated through.
7. Serve spaghetti squash topped with marinara sauce and garnish with fresh basil and Parmesan cheese if desired.

Nutrition Information:

- Calories: 180
- Protein: 4g
- Carbohydrates: 30g
- Fat: 6g
- Fiber: 8g
- Sugar: 10g
- Portion size: 1 cup spaghetti squash with sauce

Greek-Style Stuffed Tomatoes

Ingredients:

- Tomatoes
- Quinoa
- Cucumber
- Red onion
- Kalamata olives
- Feta cheese
- Lemon juice
- Olive oil
- Fresh parsley
- Salt and pepper

Instructions:

1. Cook quinoa according to package instructions and let cool.
2. Cut tops off tomatoes and scoop out seeds.
3. Dice cucumber, red onion, and olives, then mix with cooked quinoa, crumbled feta cheese, lemon juice, olive oil, chopped parsley, salt, and pepper.
4. Stuff mixture into hollowed-out tomatoes.
5. Serve chilled or at room temperature.

Nutrition Information:

- Calories: 220

- Protein: 8g

- Carbohydrates: 25g

- Fat: 10g

- Fiber: 6g

- Sugar: 8g

- Portion size: 1 stuffed tomato

Mixed Vegetable Paella

Ingredients:

- Arborio rice

- Vegetable broth

- Onion

- Garlic

- Bell peppers

- Tomatoes

- Green beans

- Artichoke hearts

- Peas

- Saffron

- Paprika

- Olive oil

- Lemon wedges (for serving)

Instructions:

1. Sauté onion and garlic in olive oil until softened.
2. Add Arborio rice and cook until translucent.
3. Stir in chopped bell peppers, diced tomatoes, sliced green beans, quartered artichoke hearts, and peas.
4. Dissolve saffron in a small amount of warm vegetable broth, then add to the rice mixture.
5. Gradually add vegetable broth, stirring occasionally, until rice is cooked through.
6. Season with paprika and salt to taste.
7. Serve hot with lemon wedges on the side.

Nutrition Information:

- Calories: 280
- Protein: 6g
- Carbohydrates: 50g
- Fat: 6g
- Fiber: 8g
- Sugar: 8g
- Portion size: 1 serving

Vegan Shepherd's Pie

Ingredients:

- Lentils
- Carrots
- Peas
- Onion
- Garlic
- Vegetable broth
- Tomato paste
- Mashed potatoes (made with non-dairy milk and vegan butter)
- Nutritional yeast
- Thyme
- Rosemary
- Olive oil
- Salt and pepper

Instructions:

1. Sauté onion and garlic in olive oil until softened.
2. Add diced carrots and cook until slightly tender.
3. Stir in cooked lentils, peas, vegetable broth, tomato paste, nutritional yeast, thyme, rosemary, salt, and pepper.
4. Simmer until mixture thickens.

5. Transfer filling to a baking dish and top with mashed potatoes.
6. Bake until potatoes are golden brown and filling is bubbling.
7. Serve hot.

Nutrition Information:

- Calories: 320
- Protein: 10g
- Carbohydrates: 40g
- Fat: 12g
- Fiber: 10g
- Sugar: 8g
- Portion size: 1 serving

Chickpea and Spinach Stew

Ingredients:

- Chickpeas
- Spinach
- Onion
- Garlic
- Tomatoes
- Vegetable broth
- Cumin

- Paprika

- Cayenne pepper

- Lemon juice

- Olive oil

- Salt and pepper

Instructions:

1. Sauté onion and garlic in olive oil until translucent.

2. Add diced tomatoes, drained chickpeas, vegetable broth, cumin, paprika, and cayenne pepper.

3. Simmer for 15-20 minutes, until flavors are well combined.

4. Stir in fresh spinach until wilted.

5. Finish with a squeeze of lemon juice and season with salt and pepper to taste.

6. Serve hot, optionally garnished with fresh parsley.

Nutrition Information:

- Calories: 250

- Protein: 10g

- Carbohydrates: 35g

- Fat: 8g

- Fiber: 10g

- Sugar: 8g

- Portion size: 1 serving

Baked Tofu with Steamed Vegetables

Ingredients:

- Tofu
- Broccoli
- Carrots
- Snap peas
- Red bell pepper
- Garlic
- Ginger
- Soy sauce
- Rice vinegar
- Sesame oil
- Olive oil
- Sesame seeds
- Green onions

Instructions:

1. Press tofu to remove excess moisture, then cut into cubes.
2. Toss tofu with soy sauce, rice vinegar, minced garlic, minced ginger, and sesame oil.
3. Arrange tofu on a baking sheet and bake at 400°F (200°C) for 20-25 minutes, until golden brown.
4. Steam broccoli, carrots, snap peas, and red bell pepper until tender-crisp.

5. Serve baked tofu with steamed vegetables, garnished with sesame seeds and chopped green onions.

Nutrition Information:

- Calories: 280
- Protein: 15g
- Carbohydrates: 20g
- Fat: 15g
- Fiber: 8g
- Sugar: 6g
- Portion size: 1 serving

Chapter 5: Snacks and Appetizers

In between meals or for entertaining guests, having a selection of nutritious snacks and appetizers is essential. These recipes are not only delicious but also packed with wholesome ingredients to keep you satisfied and energized throughout the day.

Hummus and Veggie Sticks

Ingredients:

- 1 can chickpeas, drained and rinsed
- 2 tablespoons tahini
- 2 cloves garlic, minced
- 2 tablespoons lemon juice
- 2 tablespoons olive oil
- Salt and pepper to taste
- Assorted vegetables for dipping (carrots, cucumber, bell peppers, etc.)

Instructions:

1. In a food processor, combine chickpeas, tahini, garlic, lemon juice, and olive oil.
2. Blend until smooth, adding water as needed to achieve desired consistency.

3. Season with salt and pepper to taste.

4. Serve with sliced vegetables for dipping.

Nutrition Information:

- Calories: 120
- Protein: 5g
- Carbohydrates: 14g
- Fat: 6g
- Fiber: 4g
- Sugar: 2g
- Portion size: 2 tablespoons hummus with 1 cup sliced vegetables

Roasted Chickpeas

Ingredients:

- 1 can chickpeas, drained and rinsed
- 1 tablespoon olive oil
- 1 teaspoon cumin
- 1 teaspoon paprika
- Salt to taste

Instructions:

1. Preheat oven to 400°F (200°C).

2. Pat chickpeas dry with a paper towel and place on a baking sheet.

3. Drizzle with olive oil and sprinkle with cumin, paprika, and salt.

4. Toss to coat evenly.

5. Roast in the oven for 25-30 minutes, or until crispy.

6. Allow to cool before serving.

Nutrition Information:

- Calories: 130
- Protein: 6g
- Carbohydrates: 20g
- Fat: 3g
- Fiber: 6g
- Sugar: 4g
- Portion size: 1/2 cup

Stuffed Mini Bell Peppers

Ingredients:

- 10 mini bell peppers, halved and seeds removed
- 1 cup cooked quinoa
- 1/2 cup black beans, drained and rinsed
- 1/2 cup corn kernels

- 1/4 cup diced tomatoes

- 1/4 cup diced red onion

- 1/4 cup chopped cilantro

- Juice of 1 lime

- Salt and pepper to taste

Instructions:

1. In a large bowl, mix together cooked quinoa, black beans, corn, tomatoes, red onion, cilantro, and lime juice.
2. Season with salt and pepper to taste.
3. Spoon the mixture into the halved mini bell peppers.
4. Serve chilled or at room temperature.

Nutrition Information:

- Calories: 45

- Protein: 2g

- Carbohydrates: 9g

- Fat: 0.5g

- Fiber: 2g

- Sugar: 2g

- Portion size: 2 stuffed pepper halves

Edamame with Sea Salt

Ingredients:

- 2 cups edamame, cooked and shelled
- Sea salt to taste

Instructions:

1. Steam or boil the edamame according to package instructions.
2. Drain and transfer to a serving bowl.
3. Sprinkle with sea salt to taste.
4. Toss to coat evenly.

Nutrition Information:

- Calories: 120
- Protein: 12g
- Carbohydrates: 8g
- Fat: 5g
- Fiber: 4g
- Sugar: 2g
- Portion size: 1 cup

Spicy Avocado Dip with Whole Grain Crackers

Ingredients:

- 2 ripe avocados, peeled and pitted
- 1 jalapeno, seeded and chopped
- 1/4 cup chopped cilantro
- Juice of 1 lime
- Salt and pepper to taste
- Whole grain crackers for serving

Instructions:

1. In a bowl, mash the avocados with a fork until smooth.
2. Stir in chopped jalapeno, cilantro, and lime juice.
3. Season with salt and pepper to taste.
4. Serve with whole grain crackers.

Nutrition Information:

- Calories: 150
- Protein: 2g
- Carbohydrates: 9g
- Fat: 12g
- Fiber: 7g
- Sugar: 1g
- Portion size: 1/4 cup dip with 5 crackers

Cucumber and Tomato Salad

Ingredients:

- 2 cucumbers, diced
- 2 tomatoes, diced
- 1/4 cup diced red onion
- 2 tablespoons chopped fresh parsley
- 1 tablespoon olive oil
- 1 tablespoon red wine vinegar
- Salt and pepper to taste

Instructions:

1. In a large bowl, combine diced cucumbers, tomatoes, red onion, and parsley.
2. Drizzle with olive oil and red wine vinegar.
3. Season with salt and pepper to taste.
4. Toss to coat evenly.
5. Serve chilled.

Nutrition Information:

- Calories: 60
- Protein: 2g
- Carbohydrates: 8g
- Fat: 3g
- Fiber: 2g

- Sugar: 4g

- Portion size: 1 cup salad

Greek Yogurt with Honey and Nuts

Ingredients:

- 1 cup Greek yogurt

- 1 tablespoon honey

- 2 tablespoons chopped mixed nuts (almonds, walnuts, pistachios)

Instructions:

1. In a serving bowl, spoon Greek yogurt.

2. Drizzle with honey.

3. Sprinkle chopped mixed nuts on top.

4. Serve immediately.

Nutrition Information:

- Calories: 200

- Protein: 20g

- Carbohydrates: 15g

- Fat: 8g

- Fiber: 1g

- Sugar: 12g

- Portion size: 1 cup

Baked Zucchini Chips

Ingredients:

- 2 medium zucchinis, thinly sliced
- 1 tablespoon olive oil
- 1/4 cup grated Parmesan cheese
- 1/2 teaspoon garlic powder
- Salt and pepper to taste

Instructions:

1. Preheat oven to 425°F (220°C). Line a baking sheet with parchment paper.
2. In a large bowl, toss zucchini slices with olive oil, Parmesan cheese, garlic powder, salt, and pepper.
3. Arrange zucchini slices in a single layer on the prepared baking sheet.
4. Bake for 15-20 minutes, or until golden brown and crispy.
5. Allow to cool before serving.

Nutrition Information:

- Calories: 120
- Protein: 6g

- Carbohydrates: 8g
- Fat: 7g
- Fiber: 2g
- Sugar: 4g
- Portion size: 1/2 cup

Cauliflower Buffalo Bites

Ingredients:

- 1 head cauliflower, cut into florets
- 1/2 cup whole wheat flour
- 1/2 cup unsweetened almond milk
- 1 teaspoon garlic powder
- 1 teaspoon paprika
- 1/2 cup hot sauce
- 1 tablespoon melted butter or vegan butter
- Celery sticks and ranch dressing for serving

Instructions:

1. Preheat oven to 450°F (230°C). Line a baking sheet with parchment paper.
2. In a bowl, whisk together whole wheat flour, almond milk, garlic powder, and paprika until smooth.

3. Dip cauliflower florets into the batter, shaking off excess, and place on the prepared baking sheet.

4. Bake for 20-25 minutes, or until crispy and golden brown.

5. In a small bowl, mix hot sauce and melted butter.

6. Toss baked cauliflower in the hot sauce mixture until evenly coated.

7. Serve with celery sticks and ranch dressing.

Nutrition Information:

- Calories: 100
- Protein: 3g
- Carbohydrates: 12g
- Fat: 4g
- Fiber: 3g
- Sugar: 3g
- Portion size: 1/2 cup

Guacamole with Jicama Sticks

Ingredients:

- 2 ripe avocados, peeled and pitted
- 1/4 cup diced red onion
- 1/4 cup diced tomatoes
- 1/4 cup chopped cilantro

- Juice of 1 lime

- Salt and pepper to taste

- Jicama sticks for serving

Instructions:

1. In a bowl, mash the avocados with a fork until smooth.

2. Stir in diced red onion, tomatoes, cilantro, and lime juice.

3. Season with salt and pepper to taste.

4. Serve with jicama sticks for dipping.

Nutrition Information:

- Calories: 160

- Protein: 2g

- Carbohydrates: 10g

- Fat: 14g

- Fiber: 7g

- Sugar: 2g

- Portion size: 1/4 cup guacamole with 1 cup jicama sticks

Cottage Cheese with Pineapple

Ingredients:

- 1/2 cup low-fat cottage cheese

- 1/2 cup diced pineapple

Instructions:

1. In a serving bowl, spoon cottage cheese.

2. Top with diced pineapple.

3. Serve chilled or at room temperature.

Nutrition Information:

- Calories: 120

- Protein: 14g

- Carbohydrates: 14g

- Fat: 2g

- Fiber: 1g

- Sugar: 10g

- Portion size: 1/2 cup

Vegan Sushi Rolls

Ingredients:

- Nori seaweed sheets

- Cooked sushi rice

- Assorted vegetables (cucumber, avocado, carrot, bell pepper)

- Soy sauce, for dipping

Instructions:

1. Place a nori seaweed sheet on a bamboo sushi mat.
2. Spread a thin layer of cooked sushi rice over the nori sheet.
3. Arrange sliced vegetables in the center of the rice.
4. Roll the sushi tightly using the bamboo mat.
5. Slice the roll into bite-sized pieces.
6. Serve with soy sauce for dipping.

Nutrition Information:

- Calories: 150
- Protein: 3g
- Carbohydrates: 30g
- Fat: 1g
- Fiber: 4g
- Sugar: 2g
- Portion size: 6 pieces

Spinach and Artichoke Dip

Ingredients:

- 1 cup frozen spinach, thawed and drained
- 1 can artichoke hearts, drained and chopped
- 1 cup Greek yogurt
- 1/4 cup grated Parmesan cheese

- 1/4 cup shredded mozzarella cheese
- 2 cloves garlic, minced
- Salt and pepper to taste
- Whole grain crackers or vegetable sticks for serving

Instructions:

1. Preheat oven to 375°F (190°C).
2. In a mixing bowl, combine thawed spinach, chopped artichoke hearts, Greek yogurt, Parmesan cheese, mozzarella cheese, and minced garlic.
3. Season with salt and pepper to taste.
4. Transfer the mixture to a baking dish.
5. Bake for 20-25 minutes, or until bubbly and golden brown on top.
6. Serve hot with whole grain crackers or vegetable sticks.

Nutrition Information:

- Calories: 120
- Protein: 10g
- Carbohydrates: 8g
- Fat: 5g
- Fiber: 2g
- Sugar: 2g
- Portion size: 1/4 cup dip with 5 crackers or vegetable sticks

Caprese Skewers

Ingredients:

- Cherry tomatoes
- Fresh mozzarella balls
- Fresh basil leaves
- Balsamic glaze
- Skewers

Instructions:

1. Thread one cherry tomato, one mozzarella ball, and one basil leaf onto each skewer.
2. Arrange skewers on a serving platter.
3. Drizzle with balsamic glaze.
4. Serve immediately.

Nutrition Information:

- Calories: 80
- Protein: 5g
- Carbohydrates: 3g
- Fat: 6g
- Fiber: 1g
- Sugar: 2g
- Portion size: 2 skewers

Almond Butter and Apple Slices

Ingredients:

- 2 tablespoons almond butter
- 1 medium apple, sliced

Instructions:

1. Spread almond butter on apple slices.
2. Serve immediately.

Nutrition Information:

- Calories: 200
- Protein: 4g
- Carbohydrates: 20g
- Fat: 12g
- Fiber: 6g
- Sugar: 14g
- Portion size: 1 medium apple with 2 tablespoons almond butter

Chapter 6: Desserts

Indulge your sweet tooth with these delightful dessert recipes that are not only delicious but also suitable for a diabetic-friendly diet. From creamy puddings to fruity sorbets and decadent brownies, there's something here to satisfy every craving without compromising your health goals.

Chia Seed Pudding with Fresh Berries

Ingredients:

- 1/4 cup chia seeds
- 1 cup almond milk
- 1 tablespoon maple syrup
- Fresh berries for topping

Instructions:

1. In a bowl, mix chia seeds, almond milk, and maple syrup.
2. Stir well and let it sit in the fridge for at least 2 hours or overnight.
3. Serve topped with fresh berries.

Nutrition Information:

- Calories: 180

- Protein: 4g

- Carbohydrates: 20g

- Fat: 9g

- Fiber: 10g

- Sugar: 6g

- Portion Size: 1 serving

Almond Flour Chocolate Chip Cookies

Ingredients:

- 1 1/2 cups almond flour

- 1/4 cup coconut oil, melted

- 1/4 cup maple syrup

- 1/2 teaspoon vanilla extract

- 1/4 cup dark chocolate chips

Instructions:

1. Preheat oven to 350°F (175°C) and line a baking sheet with parchment paper.

2. In a bowl, mix almond flour, coconut oil, maple syrup, and vanilla extract until well combined.

3. Fold in dark chocolate chips.

4. Form dough into small balls and place them on the baking sheet.

5. Flatten each ball slightly with the back of a spoon.

6. Bake for 10-12 minutes or until golden brown.

7. Let cool before serving.

Nutrition Information:

- Calories: 150
- Protein: 3g
- Carbohydrates: 10g
- Fat: 12g
- Fiber: 2g
- Sugar: 6g
- Portion Size: 2 cookies

Greek Yogurt Parfait with Mixed Berries

Ingredients:

- 1 cup Greek yogurt
- 1/2 cup mixed berries (such as strawberries, blueberries, and raspberries)
- 1 tablespoon honey or maple syrup
- 2 tablespoons granola

Instructions:

1. In a glass or bowl, layer Greek yogurt, mixed berries, and granola.
2. Drizzle honey or maple syrup over the top.
3. Repeat layers until ingredients are used up.
4. Serve immediately.

Nutrition Information:

- Calories: 200
- Protein: 15g
- Carbohydrates: 25g
- Fat: 5g
- Fiber: 3g
- Sugar: 15g
- Portion Size: 1 serving

Baked Apples with Cinnamon

Ingredients:

- 2 apples, cored and sliced
- 1 tablespoon lemon juice
- 1 teaspoon cinnamon
- 1 tablespoon maple syrup

Instructions:

1. Preheat oven to 350°F (175°C).

2. Toss apple slices with lemon juice, cinnamon, and maple syrup in a baking dish.

3. Bake for 20-25 minutes or until apples are tender.

4. Serve warm.

Nutrition Information:

- Calories: 120

- Protein: 1g

- Carbohydrates: 30g

- Fat: 0g

- Fiber: 5g

- Sugar: 20g

- Portion Size: 1/2 apple

Sugar-Free Chocolate Avocado Mousse

Ingredients:

- 2 ripe avocados

- 1/4 cup unsweetened cocoa powder

- 1/4 cup almond milk

- 2 tablespoons maple syrup or sweetener of choice

- 1 teaspoon vanilla extract

Instructions:

1. In a food processor or blender, combine avocados, cocoa powder, almond milk, maple syrup, and vanilla extract.
2. Blend until smooth and creamy, scraping down the sides as needed.
3. Transfer to serving dishes and chill in the fridge for at least 30 minutes before serving.

Nutrition Information:

- Calories: 180
- Protein: 3g
- Carbohydrates: 15g
- Fat: 14g
- Fiber: 8g
- Sugar: 4g
- Portion Size: 1/2 cup

Carrot Cake Energy Balls

Ingredients:

- 1 cup rolled oats
- 1/2 cup shredded carrots
- 1/4 cup almond butter
- 2 tablespoons maple syrup

- 1 teaspoon cinnamon

- 1/4 cup chopped walnuts

- 1/4 cup shredded coconut (optional)

Instructions:

1. In a food processor, combine rolled oats, shredded carrots, almond butter, maple syrup, and cinnamon.
2. Pulse until mixture comes together.
3. Stir in chopped walnuts and shredded coconut, if using.
4. Roll mixture into small balls and refrigerate for at least 30 minutes before serving.

Nutrition Information:

- Calories: 90
- Protein: 3g
- Carbohydrates: 10g
- Fat: 5g
- Fiber: 2g
- Sugar: 3g
- Portion Size: 2 balls

Coconut Macaroons

Ingredients:

- 2 cups shredded coconut
- 1/4 cup coconut flour
- 1/4 cup coconut oil, melted
- 1/4 cup maple syrup
- 1 teaspoon vanilla extract
- Pinch of salt

Instructions:

1. Preheat oven to 350°F (175°C) and line a baking sheet with parchment paper.
2. In a bowl, mix together shredded coconut, coconut flour, melted coconut oil, maple syrup, vanilla extract, and salt until well combined.
3. Using a tablespoon, scoop out the mixture and form into small mounds on the prepared baking sheet.
4. Bake for 10-12 minutes or until lightly golden brown.
5. Let cool completely before serving.

Nutrition Information:

- Calories: 120
- Protein: 1g
- Carbohydrates: 8g

- Fat: 10g

- Fiber: 2g

- Sugar: 5g

- Portion Size: 2 macaroons

Strawberry and Basil Sorbet

Ingredients:

- 2 cups frozen strawberries

- 1/4 cup fresh basil leaves

- 2 tablespoons honey or maple syrup

- 1 tablespoon lemon juice

Instructions:

1. In a blender, combine frozen strawberries, fresh basil leaves, honey or maple syrup, and lemon juice.

2. Blend until smooth and creamy.

3. Transfer mixture to a shallow dish and freeze for at least 2 hours, stirring every 30 minutes.

4. Serve scoops of sorbet in bowls or cones.

Nutrition Information:

- Calories: 60

- Protein: 1g

- Carbohydrates: 15g

- Fat: 0g

- Fiber: 3g

- Sugar: 10g

- Portion Size: 1/2 cup

Dark Chocolate and Nut Clusters

Ingredients:

- 1/2 cup dark chocolate chips

- 1/4 cup mixed nuts (such as almonds, walnuts, and pecans)

Instructions:

1. Melt dark chocolate chips in a microwave-safe bowl in 30-second intervals, stirring in between until smooth.

2. Stir in mixed nuts until well coated.

3. Drop spoonfuls of the mixture onto a parchment-lined baking sheet.

4. Let cool until chocolate hardens, then enjoy!

Nutrition Information:

- Calories: 120

- Protein: 2g

- Carbohydrates: 10g

- Fat: 8g

- Fiber: 2g

- Sugar: 6g

- Portion Size: 2 clusters

Vegan Blueberry Muffins

Ingredients:

- 1 1/2 cups whole wheat flour

- 1/2 cup almond flour

- 1 teaspoon baking powder

- 1/2 teaspoon baking soda

- 1/4 teaspoon salt

- 1/2 cup unsweetened applesauce

- 1/4 cup maple syrup

- 1/4 cup almond milk

- 1 teaspoon vanilla extract

- 1 cup fresh or frozen blueberries

Instructions:

1. Preheat oven to 350°F (175°C) and line a muffin tin with paper liners.

2. In a large bowl, whisk together whole wheat flour, almond flour, baking powder, baking soda, and salt.

3. In another bowl, mix together applesauce, maple syrup, almond milk, and vanilla extract.

4. Pour wet ingredients into dry ingredients and stir until just combined.

5. Gently fold in blueberries.

6. Divide batter evenly among muffin cups.

7. Bake for 20-25 minutes or until a toothpick inserted into the center comes out clean.

8. Let cool before serving.

Nutrition Information:

- Calories: 120
- Protein: 3g
- Carbohydrates: 20g
- Fat: 3g
- Fiber: 3g
- Sugar: 8g
- Portion Size: 1 muffin

Matcha Green Tea Ice Cream

Ingredients:

- 2 ripe bananas, sliced and frozen
- 1 tablespoon matcha powder

- 1/4 cup coconut milk

- 1 tablespoon honey or maple syrup (optional)

Instructions:

1. In a blender or food processor, combine frozen banana slices, matcha powder, coconut milk, and honey or maple syrup.

2. Blend until smooth and creamy, scraping down the sides as needed.

3. Transfer mixture to a freezer-safe container and freeze for at least 2 hours, or until firm.

4. Serve scoops of matcha green tea ice cream and enjoy!

Nutrition Information:

- Calories: 120

- Protein: 2g

- Carbohydrates: 25g

- Fat: 3g

- Fiber: 3g

- Sugar: 14g

- Portion Size: 1/2 cup

Lemon Chia Seed Muffins

Ingredients:

- 1 1/2 cups whole wheat flour
- 1/2 cup almond flour
- 1/4 cup chia seeds
- 1 teaspoon baking powder
- 1/2 teaspoon baking soda
- 1/4 teaspoon salt
- 1/2 cup unsweetened applesauce
- 1/4 cup maple syrup
- 1/4 cup almond milk
- 1/4 cup lemon juice
- Zest of 1 lemon

Instructions:

1. Preheat oven to 350°F (175°C) and line a muffin tin with paper liners.
2. In a large bowl, whisk together whole wheat flour, almond flour, chia seeds, baking powder, baking soda, and salt.
3. In another bowl, mix together applesauce, maple syrup, almond milk, lemon juice, and lemon zest.
4. Pour wet ingredients into dry ingredients and stir until just combined.
5. Divide batter evenly among muffin cups.

6. Bake for 20-25 minutes or until a toothpick inserted into the center comes out clean.

7. Let cool before serving.

Nutrition Information:

- Calories: 130

- Protein: 3g

- Carbohydrates: 22g

- Fat: 4g

- Fiber: 4g

- Sugar: 6g

- Portion Size: 1 muffin

Banana Nice Cream

Ingredients:

- 2 ripe bananas, sliced and frozen

- 2 tablespoons almond milk (or any milk of choice)

- 1 teaspoon vanilla extract

- Toppings of choice (such as chopped nuts, shredded coconut, or dark chocolate chips)

Instructions:

1. In a blender or food processor, blend frozen banana slices, almond milk, and vanilla extract until smooth and creamy.
2. Transfer the mixture to a bowl.
3. Serve immediately as soft-serve ice cream or freeze for 30 minutes for a firmer texture.
4. Top with your favorite toppings and enjoy!

Nutrition Information:

- Calories: 100
- Protein: 1g
- Carbohydrates: 25g
- Fat: 1g
- Fiber: 3g
- Sugar: 14g
- Portion Size: 1/2 cup

Pumpkin Pie Bites

Ingredients:

- 1 cup pumpkin puree
- 1/4 cup almond flour
- 2 tablespoons maple syrup
- 1 teaspoon pumpkin pie spice

- 1/4 cup chopped pecans

Instructions:

1. In a bowl, mix together pumpkin puree, almond flour, maple syrup, and pumpkin pie spice until well combined.
2. Roll the mixture into small balls and place them on a baking sheet lined with parchment paper.
3. Press a chopped pecan into the top of each ball.
4. Chill in the fridge for at least 30 minutes before serving.

Nutrition Information:

- Calories: 80
- Protein: 2g
- Carbohydrates: 8g
- Fat: 5g
- Fiber: 2g
- Sugar: 4g
- Portion Size: 2 bites

Raw Vegan Brownies

Ingredients:

- 1 cup Medjool dates, pitted
- 1 cup walnuts

- 1/4 cup unsweetened cocoa powder
- Pinch of salt

Instructions:

1. Place dates and walnuts in a food processor and blend until finely chopped and well combined.
2. Add cocoa powder and salt to the mixture and blend again until a sticky dough forms.
3. Press the dough into a lined baking dish or pan.
4. Chill in the fridge for at least 1 hour before cutting into squares and serving.

Nutrition Information:

- Calories: 120
- Protein: 2g
- Carbohydrates: 15g
- Fat: 7g
- Fiber: 3g
- Sugar: 11g
- Portion Size: 1 brownie square

Chapter 7: Smoothies

These refreshing and nutritious drinks are perfect for a quick breakfast, post-workout snack, or anytime pick-me-up. Packed with vitamins, minerals, and antioxidants, these smoothie recipes will keep you energized and satisfied throughout the day.

Green Detox Smoothie

Ingredients:

- 1 cup spinach
- 1/2 cucumber, peeled
- 1/2 green apple, cored
- 1/2 banana
- 1/2 lemon, juiced
- 1 cup water or coconut water
- Ice cubes (optional)

Instructions:

1. Place all ingredients in a blender.
2. Blend until smooth.
3. Serve immediately and enjoy!

Nutrition Information:

- Calories: 120
- Protein: 3g
- Carbohydrates: 27g
- Fat: 1g
- Fiber: 6g
- Sugar: 15g
- Portion size: 1 smoothie

Berry Blast Smoothie

Ingredients:

- 1/2 cup mixed berries (strawberries, blueberries, raspberries)
- 1/2 banana
- 1/2 cup plain Greek yogurt
- 1/2 cup almond milk
- 1 tablespoon honey or maple syrup (optional)
- Ice cubes (optional)

Instructions:

1. Combine all ingredients in a blender.
2. Blend until smooth and creamy.
3. Pour into a glass and enjoy!

Nutrition Information:

- Calories: 180
- Protein: 10g
- Carbohydrates: 30g
- Fat: 3g
- Fiber: 5g
- Sugar: 20g
- Portion size: 1 smoothie

Tropical Mango Smoothie

Ingredients:

- 1 cup frozen mango chunks
- 1/2 banana
- 1/2 cup coconut milk
- 1/2 cup pineapple chunks
- 1/2 cup orange juice
- Ice cubes (optional)

Instructions:

1. In a blender, combine all the ingredients.
2. Blend until smooth and creamy.
3. Pour into a glass and serve immediately.

Nutrition Information:

- Calories: 200
- Protein: 2g
- Carbohydrates: 40g
- Fat: 5g
- Fiber: 4g
- Sugar: 30g
- Portion size: 1 smoothie

Peanut Butter Banana Smoothie

Ingredients:

- 1 banana
- 2 tablespoons peanut butter
- 1 cup almond milk
- 1 tablespoon honey or maple syrup (optional)
- Ice cubes (optional)

Instructions:

1. Peel the banana and place it in a blender.
2. Add the peanut butter, almond milk, and honey or maple syrup if using.
3. Blend until smooth and creamy.
4. Pour into a glass and enjoy!

Nutrition Information:

- Calories: 280
- Protein: 8g
- Carbohydrates: 30g
- Fat: 16g
- Fiber: 4g
- Sugar: 18g
- Portion size: 1 smoothie

Spinach and Pineapple Smoothie

Ingredients:

- 1 cup fresh spinach
- 1 cup pineapple chunks
- 1/2 banana
- 1/2 cup Greek yogurt
- 1/2 cup coconut water
- Ice cubes (optional)

Instructions:

1. Place all ingredients in a blender.
2. Blend until smooth and creamy.
3. Pour into a glass and enjoy!

Nutrition Information:

- Calories: 160
- Protein: 7g
- Carbohydrates: 30g
- Fat: 1g
- Fiber: 4g
- Sugar: 20g
- Portion size: 1 smoothie

Almond Berry Smoothie

Ingredients:

- 1/2 cup mixed berries (strawberries, blueberries, raspberries)
- 1/2 cup almond milk
- 1/4 cup plain Greek yogurt
- 1 tablespoon almond butter
- 1 tablespoon honey or maple syrup (optional)
- Ice cubes (optional)

Instructions:

1. Combine all ingredients in a blender.
2. Blend until smooth and creamy.
3. Pour into a glass and serve immediately.

Nutrition Information:

- Calories: 200
- Protein: 8g
- Carbohydrates: 25g
- Fat: 8g
- Fiber: 5g
- Sugar: 15g
- Portion size: 1 smoothie

Cucumber Mint Smoothie

Ingredients:

- 1 cucumber, peeled and chopped
- 1/4 cup fresh mint leaves
- 1/2 cup spinach
- 1/2 cup plain Greek yogurt
- 1/2 cup coconut water
- Juice of 1 lime
- Ice cubes (optional)

Instructions:

1. Place all ingredients in a blender.
2. Blend until smooth and creamy.
3. Pour into a glass and enjoy!

Nutrition Information:

- Calories: 120
- Protein: 8g
- Carbohydrates: 20g
- Fat: 2g
- Fiber: 4g
- Sugar: 12g
- Portion size: 1 smoothie

Avocado Lime Smoothie

Ingredients:

- 1 ripe avocado
- Juice of 2 limes
- 1 cup spinach
- 1/2 cup almond milk
- 1 tablespoon honey or maple syrup (optional)
- Ice cubes (optional)

Instructions:

1. Scoop the avocado flesh into a blender.
2. Add lime juice, spinach, almond milk, and honey or maple syrup if using.
3. Blend until smooth and creamy.

4. Serve immediately.

Nutrition Information:

- Calories: 220
- Protein: 4g
- Carbohydrates: 20g
- Fat: 15g
- Fiber: 8g
- Sugar: 8g
- Portion size: 1 smoothie

Chocolate Protein Smoothie

Ingredients:

- 1 scoop chocolate protein powder
- 1 banana
- 1 tablespoon almond butter
- 1 cup almond milk
- Ice cubes (optional)

Instructions:

1. Place all ingredients in a blender.
2. Blend until smooth and creamy.
3. Pour into a glass and enjoy!

Nutrition Information:

- Calories: 300
- Protein: 25g
- Carbohydrates: 30g
- Fat: 10g
- Fiber: 5g
- Sugar: 15g
- Portion size: 1 smoothie

Carrot Ginger Smoothie

Ingredients:

- 1 carrot, peeled and chopped
- 1/2 inch piece of fresh ginger, peeled
- 1/2 banana
- 1/2 cup orange juice
- 1/2 cup Greek yogurt
- Ice cubes (optional)

Instructions:

1. Place all ingredients in a blender.
2. Blend until smooth and creamy.
3. Pour into a glass and enjoy!

Nutrition Information:

- Calories: 140
- Protein: 6g
- Carbohydrates: 30g
- Fat: 1g
- Fiber: 3g
- Sugar: 20g
- Portion size: 1 smoothie

Apple Cinnamon Smoothie

Ingredients:

- 1 apple, cored and chopped
- 1/2 teaspoon ground cinnamon
- 1/2 cup plain Greek yogurt
- 1/2 cup almond milk
- 1 tablespoon honey or maple syrup (optional)
- Ice cubes (optional)

Instructions:

1. Combine all ingredients in a blender.
2. Blend until smooth and creamy.
3. Pour into a glass and serve immediately.

Nutrition Information:

- Calories: 180
- Protein: 8g
- Carbohydrates: 30g
- Fat: 3g
- Fiber: 5g
- Sugar: 20g
- Portion size: 1 smoothie

Strawberry Banana Smoothie

Ingredients:

- 1/2 cup strawberries, hulled
- 1 banana
- 1/2 cup plain Greek yogurt
- 1/2 cup almond milk
- 1 tablespoon honey or maple syrup (optional)
- Ice cubes (optional)

Instructions:

1. Place all ingredients in a blender.
2. Blend until smooth and creamy.
3. Pour into a glass and enjoy!

Nutrition Information:

- Calories: 200
- Protein: 9g
- Carbohydrates: 35g
- Fat: 2g
- Fiber: 6g
- Sugar: 25g
- Portion size: 1 smoothie

Blueberry Oat Smoothie

Ingredients:

- 1/2 cup blueberries
- 1/4 cup rolled oats
- 1/2 banana
- 1/2 cup almond milk
- 1/2 cup plain Greek yogurt
- 1 tablespoon honey or maple syrup (optional)
- Ice cubes (optional)

Instructions:

1. Combine all ingredients in a blender.
2. Blend until smooth and creamy.
3. Pour into a glass and serve immediately.

Nutrition Information:

- Calories: 220
- Protein: 10g
- Carbohydrates: 35g
- Fat: 4g
- Fiber: 5g
- Sugar: 20g
- Portion size: 1 smoothie

Coconut Water and Berry Smoothie

Ingredients:

- 1/2 cup mixed berries (strawberries, blueberries, raspberries)
- 1/2 cup coconut water
- 1/2 cup plain Greek yogurt
- 1 tablespoon honey or maple syrup (optional)
- Ice cubes (optional)

Instructions:

1. Place all ingredients in a blender.
2. Blend until smooth and creamy.
3. Pour into a glass and enjoy!

Nutrition Information:

- Calories: 180
- Protein: 8g
- Carbohydrates: 30g
- Fat: 2g
- Fiber: 5g
- Sugar: 20g
- Portion size: 1 smoothie

Kiwi and Kale Smoothie

Ingredients:

- 2 kiwis, peeled and chopped
- 1 cup chopped kale leaves
- 1/2 banana
- 1/2 cup almond milk
- 1/2 cup plain Greek yogurt
- 1 tablespoon honey or maple syrup (optional)
- Ice cubes (optional)

Instructions:

1. Place all ingredients in a blender.
2. Blend until smooth and creamy.
3. Pour into a glass and serve immediately.

Nutrition Information:

- Calories: 200
- Protein: 9g
- Carbohydrates: 35g
- Fat: 3g
- Fiber: 7g
- Sugar: 20g
- Portion size: 1 smoothie

CONCLUSION

Throughout this journey, you've explored the intersection of diabetes management and vegetarianism, discovering a rich array of flavorful and nutritious recipes carefully curated to support your dietary needs and preferences.

As you've navigated through the 30-day meal plan, relished in breakfast delights, savored satisfying lunches, indulged in wholesome dinners, and enjoyed guilt-free snacks and desserts, you've empowered yourself with knowledge and practical tools for sustainable dietary habits.

Remember, this journey is not just about what you eat but also about embracing a lifestyle that nourishes both body and soul. By prioritizing whole foods, fiber-rich ingredients, and mindful eating practices, you're not just managing your diabetes – you're thriving.

As you bid farewell to these pages, carry with you the confidence and inspiration to continue exploring the endless possibilities of diabetic-friendly vegetarian cuisine. Whether you're embarking on this journey for health reasons, ethical beliefs, or simply a love for vibrant flavors, know that each meal is a celebration of life and a step towards a brighter, healthier future.

Here's to your health, happiness, and culinary adventures ahead. Cheers to a lifetime of delicious, diabetes-friendly meals!